Mediterranean Diet Cookbook

The best guide to your air fryer delicious recipes
Smoothies and Salad

Michelle Burns

Table of Contents

1 . ONION-MUSHROOM OMELET...1

2 . SCRAMBLED EGGS WITH VEGETABLES 3

3 . CITRUS GREEN JUICE...5

4 . PANCETTA & EGG BENEDICT WITH ARUGULA 7

5 . CHILI ZUCCHINI & EGG NESTS....................................9

6 . PEACH & PECAN PARFAIT 11

7 . CHIA & BANANA OATS 13

8 . AVOCADO EGG SCRAMBLE 15

9 . PARMESAN OMELET 17

10 . WATERMELON PIZZA..19

11 . MORNING PIZZA WITH SPROUTS 21

12 . AVOCADO MILK SHAKE 23

13 . CAULIFLOWER FRITTERS 25

14 . BAKED OATMEAL WITH CINNAMON...........................27

15 . COCOA OATMEAL 29

16 . PUMPKIN OATMEAL WITH SPICES 31

17 . BREAKFAST SPANAKOPITA 33

18 . OVERNIGHT OATS WITH NUTS...................................35

19 . POBLANO FRITATTA 37

20 . VEGETABLE BREAKFAST BOWL 39

21 . SIMPLE AND QUICK STEAK 41

22 . CHEESY EGGS IN AVOCADO 43

23 . FOUR-CHEESE ZUCCHINI NOODLES WITH BASIL PESTO 45

24 . HEAVENLY EGG BAKE WITH BLACKBERRY 47

25 . BLUEBERRY AND VANILLA SCONES 49

26 . AVOCADO AND EGGS BREAKFAST TACOS..................51

27 . AWESOME COFFEE WITH BUTTER 53

28 . CHEESY CAPRESE STYLE PORTOBELLOS MUSHROOMS 55

29 . SCRAMBLED EGGS 57

30 . CREAMY PARSLEY SOUFFLÉ... 59

31 . SPINACH ARTICHOKE EGG CASSEROLE 61

32 . CINNAMON FAUX-ST CRUNCH CEREAL................................. 63

33 . KETO EGG FAST SNICKERDOODLE CREPES 65

34 . OAT & CARROT CUPCAKES 67

35 . MUSHROOM & CHERRY TOMATO FRITTATA 69

36 . STRAWBERRY-CHOCOLATE SMOOTHIE 71

37 . YOGURT PARFAIT WITH BERRIES & GRANOLA 73

38 . CHEESY CAULIFLOWER FRITTATA 75

39 . COCONUT & CHOCOLATE PORRIDGE WITH BANANAS 77

40 . CILANTRO MOZZARELLA & OLIVE CAKES 79

41 . CHEDDAR EGG SANDWICH WITH VEGGIES 81

42 . MUSHROOM & QUINOA CUPS... 83

43 . RASPBERRY OAT PUDDING 85

44 . CLASSIC SPANISH TORTILLA 87

45 . ONION-MUSHROOM OMELET 89

46 . ZUCCHINI & MUSHROOM EGG CAKES.................................. 91

47 . EGG & ZUCCHINI STUFFED TOMATOES 93

48 . ANCHOVY EGG SCRAMBLE... 95

49 . WATERCRESS & EGG SALAD WITH QUINOA 97

50 . VEGETABLE EGG BAKE 99

51 . AWESOME TUNA SALAD..101

52 . SHRIMP & AVOCADO SALAD...103

53 . ONE-PAN EGGPLANT QUINOA 105

54 . ARUGULA & GORGONZOLA SALAD 107

55 . GREEK-STYLE PASTA SALAD...109

56 . CHEESY THYME WAFFLES **111**

57 . LOW CARB GREEN SMOOTHIE **113**

1. Onion-Mushroom Omelet

INGREDIENTS (2 Servings)

- 4 eggs, beaten
- 1 cup mushrooms sliced
- 2 tsp olive oil,
- divided 1 garlic clove,
- minced Salt and black pepper to taste
- ¼ cup sliced onions

DIRECTIONS (15 minutes)

Warm the olive oil in a frying pan over medium heat. Place in garlic, mushrooms, and onions. Cook for 6 minutes, stirring often. Season with salt and pepper. Increase the heat and cook for 3 minutes. Remove to a plate. In the same pan, add in the eggs and ensure they are evenly spread. Top with the veggies. Slice into wedges and serve.

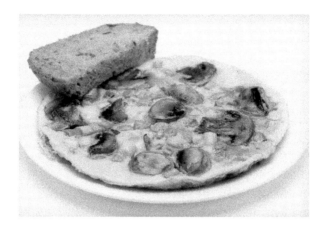

Notes:

2. Scrambled Eggs with Vegetables

INGREDIENTS (4 Servings)

- 6 cherry tomatoes,
- halved 2 tbsp olive oil
- ½ cup chopped zucchini
- ½ cup chopped green bell pepper
- 8 eggs, beaten
- 1 shallot, chopped
- 1 tbsp chopped fresh parsley
- 1 tbsp chopped fresh basil
- Salt and black pepper to taste

DIRECTIONS (15 minutes)

Warm oil in a pan over medium heat. Place in zucchini, salt, black pepper and shallot. Cook for 4-5 minutes to sweat the shallot. Stir in tomatoes, parsley, and basil. Cook for a minute and top with the beaten eggs. Lower the heat and cook for 6-7 minutes until the eggs are set but not runny. Remove to a platter to serve.

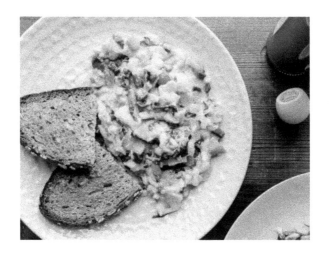

Notes:

3. Citrus Green Juice

- ½ grapefruit
- ½ lemon
- 3 cups cavolo nero
- 1 cucumber
- ¼ cup fresh parsley leaves
- ¼ pineapple, cut into wedges
- ½ green apple
- 1 tsp grated fresh ginger

DIRECTIONS (5 minutes)

In a mixer, place the cavolo nero, parsley, cucumber, pineapple, grapefruit, apple, lemon, and ginger and pulse until smooth. Serve in a tall glass.

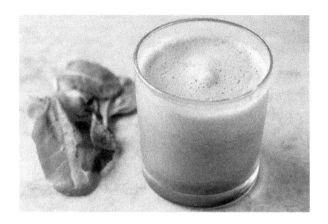

Notes:

4. Pancetta & Egg Benedict with Arugula

INGREDIENTS (2 Servings)

- 1 English muffin,
- toasted and halved
- ¼ cup chopped pancetta
- 2 tsp hollandaise sauce
- 1 cup arugula
- Salt and black pepper to taste
- 2 large eggs

DIRECTIONS (20 minutes)

Place pancetta in a pan over medium heat and cook for 5 minutes until crispy. Remove to a bowl. In the same pan, crack the eggs and season with salt and pepper. Cook for 4-5 minutes until the whites are set. Turn the eggs and cook for an additional minute. Divide pancetta between muffin halves and top each with an egg. Spoon the hollandaise sauce on top and sprinkle with arugula to serve.

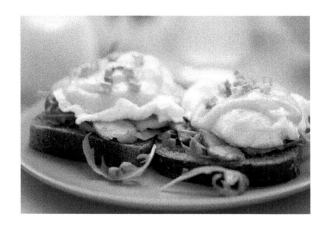

Notes:

5. Chili Zucchini & Egg Nests

- 4 eggs
- 2 tbsp olive oil
- 1 lb zucchinis,
- shredded Salt and black pepper to taste
- ½ red chili pepper,
- seeded and minced
- 2 tbsp parsley, chopped

DIRECTIONS (25 minutes)

Preheat the oven to 360 F. Combine zucchini, salt, pepper, and olive oil in a bowl. Form nest shapes with a spoon onto a greased baking sheet. Crack an egg into each nest and season with salt, pepper, and chili pepper. Bake for 11 minutes. Serve topped with parsley.

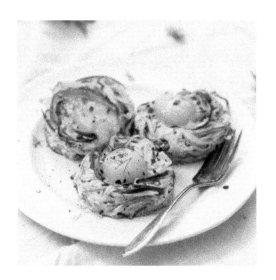

Notes:

6. Peach & Pecan Parfait

INGREDIENTS (2 Servings)

- 1 ½ cups Greek yogurt
- ½ cup pecans
- ½ cup whole-grain rolled oats
- 1 tsp honey
- 1 peeled and chopped peach
- Mint leaves for garnish

DIRECTIONS (15 minutes)

Preheat oven to 310 F. Pour the oats and pecans in a baking sheet and spread evenly. Toast for 11-13 minutes; set aside. Microwave honey for 30 seconds. Stir in the peach. Divide some of the peach mixture between 2 glasses, spread some yogurt on top, and sprinkle with the oat mixture. Repeat the layering process to exhaust the ingredients, finishing with a peach mixture. Serve with mint leaves.

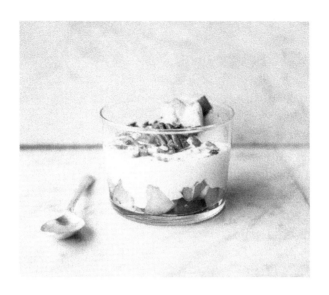

Notes:

7. Chia & Banana Oats

- ½ cup walnuts,
- chopped
- 1 banana,
- peeled and sliced
- 1 cup Greek yogurt
- 2 dates, pitted and chopped
- 1 cup rolled oats
- 2 tbsp chia seeds

DIRECTIONS (10 minutes)

Place banana, yogurt, dates, cocoa powder, oats, and chia seeds in a bowl and blend until smooth. Let sit for 1 hour and spoon onto bowl. Sprinkle with walnuts and serve.

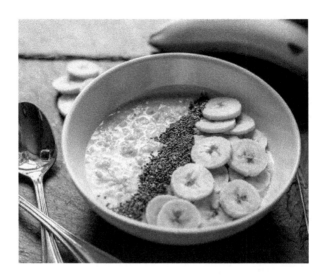

Notes:

8. Avocado Egg Scramble

- 4 eggs, beaten
- 1 white onion, diced
- 1 tablespoon avocado oil
- 1 avocado, finely chopped
- ½ teaspoon chili flakes
- 1 oz Cheddar cheese, shredded
- ½ teaspoon salt
- 1 tablespoon fresh parsley

DIRECTIONS (23 minutes)

Pour avocado oil in the skillet and bring it to boil. Then add diced onion and roast it until it is light brown. Meanwhile, mix up together chili flakes, beaten eggs, and salt. Pour the egg mixture over the cooked onion and cook the mixture for 1 minute over the medium heat. After this, scramble the eggs well with the help of the fork or spatula. Cook the eggs until they are solid but soft. After this, add chopped avocado and shredded cheese. Stir the scramble well and transfer in the serving plates. Sprinkle the meal with fresh parsley.

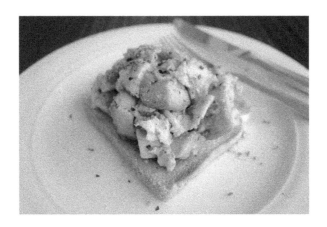

Notes:

9. Parmesan Omelet

- 1 tablespoon cream cheese
- 2 eggs, beaten
- ¼ teaspoon paprika
- ½ teaspoon dried oregano
- ¼ teaspoon dried dill
- 1 oz Parmesan, grated
- 1 teaspoon coconut oil

Mix up together cream cheese with eggs, dried oregano, and dill. Place coconut oil in the skillet and heat it up until it will coat all the skillet. Then pour the egg mixture in the skillet and flatten it. Add grated Parmesan and close the lid. Cook omelet for 10 minutes over the low heat. Then transfer the cooked omelet in the serving plate and sprinkle with paprika.

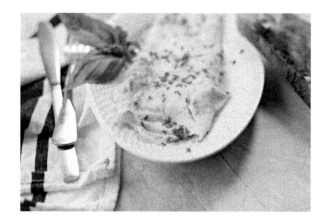

Notes:

10. Watermelon Pizza

INGREDIENTS (2 Servings)

- 9 oz watermelon slice
- 1 tablespoon Pomegranate sauce
- 2 oz Feta cheese, crumbled
- 1 tablespoon fresh cilantro, chopped

DIRECTIONS (10 minutes)

Place the watermelon slice in the plate and sprinkle with crumbled Feta cheese. Add fresh cilantro. After this, sprinkle the pizza with Pomegranate juice generously. Cut the pizza into the servings.

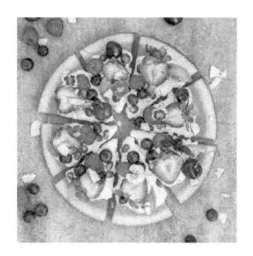

Notes:

11. Morning Pizza with Sprouts

- ½ cup wheat flour, whole grain
- 2 tablespoons butter, softened
- ¼ teaspoon baking powder
- ¾ teaspoon salt
- 5 oz chicken fillet, boiled
- 2 oz Cheddar cheese, shredded
- 1 teaspoon tomato sauce
- 1 oz bean sprouts

DIRECTIONS (35 minutes)

Make the pizza crust: mix up together wheat flour, butter, baking powder, and salt. Knead the soft and non-sticky dough. Add more wheat flour if needed. Leave the dough for 10 minutes to chill. Then place the dough on the baking paper. Cover it with the second baking paper sheet. Roll up the dough with the help of the rolling pin to get the round pizza crust. After this, remove the upper baking paper sheet. Transfer the pizza crust in the tray. Spread the crust with tomato sauce. Then shred the chicken fillet and arrange it over the pizza crust. Add shredded Cheddar cheese. Bake pizza for 20 minutes at 355F. Then top the cooked pizza with bean sprouts and slice into the servings.

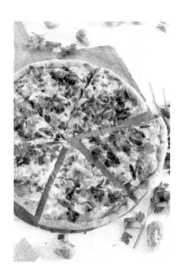

Notes:

12. Avocado Milk Shake

INGREDIENTS (3 Servings)

- 1 avocado, peeled, pitted
- 2 tablespoons of liquid honey
- ½ teaspoon vanilla extract
- ½ cup heavy cream
- 1 cup milk
- 1/3 cup ice cubes

DIRECTIONS (10 minutes)

Chop the avocado and put in the food processor. Add liquid honey, vanilla extract, heavy cream, milk, and ice cubes. Blend the mixture until it smooth. Pour the cooked milkshake in the serving glasses.

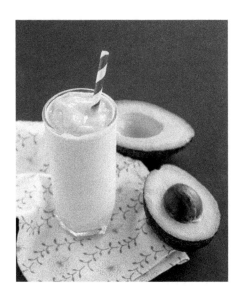

Notes:

13. Cauliflower Fritters

- 1 cup cauliflower, shredded
- 1 egg, beaten
- 1 tablespoon wheat flour, whole grain
- 1 oz Parmesan, grated
- ½ teaspoon ground black pepper
- 1 tablespoon canola oil

DIRECTIONS (20 minutes)

In the mixing bowl mix up together shredded cauliflower and egg. Add wheat flour, grated Parmesan, and ground black pepper. Stir the mixture with the help of the fork until it is homogenous and smooth. Pour canola oil in the skillet and bring it to boil. Make the fritters from the cauliflower mixture with the help of the fingertips or use spoon and transfer in the hot oil. Roast the fritters for 4 minutes from each side over the medium-low heat.

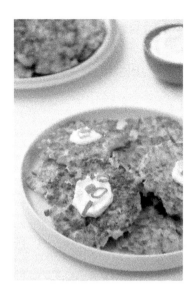

Notes:

14. Baked Oatmeal with Cinnamon

INGREDIENTS (4 Servings)

- 1 cup oatmeal
- 1/3 cup milk
- 1 pear, chopped
- 1 teaspoon vanilla extract
- 1 tablespoon Splenda
- 1 teaspoon butter
- ½ teaspoon ground cinnamon
- 1 egg, beaten

DIRECTIONS (35 minutes)

In the big bowl mix up together oatmeal, milk, egg, vanilla extract, Splenda, and ground cinnamon. Melt butter and add it in the oatmeal mixture. Then add chopped pear and stir it well. Transfer the oatmeal mixture in the casserole mold and flatten gently. Cover it with the foil and secure edges. Bake the oatmeal for 25 minutes at 350F.

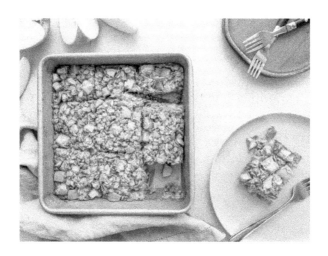

Notes:

15. Cocoa Oatmeal

- 1 ½ cup oatmeal
- 1 tablespoon cocoa powder
- ½ cup heavy cream
- ¼ cup of water
- 1 teaspoon vanilla extract
- 1 tablespoon butter
- 2 tablespoons Splenda

DIRECTIONS (25 minutes)

Mix up together oatmeal with cocoa powder and Splenda. Transfer the mixture in the saucepan. Add vanilla extract, water, and heavy cream. Stir it gently with the help of the spatula. Close the lid and cook it for 10-15 minutes over the medium-low heat. Remove the cooked cocoa oatmeal from the heat and add butter. Stir it well.

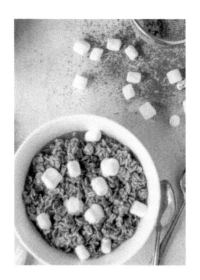

Notes:

16. Pumpkin Oatmeal with Spices

INGREDIENTS (6 Servings)

- 2 cups oatmeal
- 1 cup of coconut milk
- 1 cup milk
- 1 teaspoon Pumpkin pie spices
- 2 tablespoons pumpkin puree
- 1 tablespoon Honey
- ½ teaspoon butter

DIRECTIONS (23 minutes)

Pour coconut milk and milk in the saucepan. Add butter and bring the liquid to boil. Add oatmeal, stir well with the help of a spoon and close the lid. Simmer the oatmeal for 7 minutes over the medium heat. Meanwhile, mix up together honey, pumpkin pie spices, and pumpkin puree. When the oatmeal is cooked, add pumpkin puree mixture and stir well. Transfer the cooked breakfast in the serving plates.

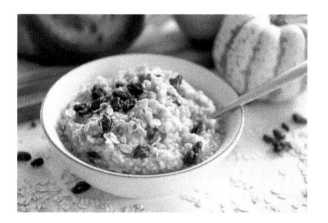

Notes:

17. Breakfast Spanakopita

INGREDIENTS (6 Servings)

- 2 cups spinach
- 1 white onion, diced
- ½ cup fresh parsley
- 1 teaspoon minced garlic
- 3 oz Feta cheese, crumbled
- 1 teaspoon ground paprika
- 2 eggs, beaten
- 1/3 cup butter, melted
- 2 oz Phyllo dough

DIRECTIONS (1 hour 15 minutes)

Separate Phyllo dough into 2 parts. Brush the casserole mold with butter well and place 1 part of Phyllo dough inside. Brush its surface with butter too. Put the spinach and fresh parsley in the blender. Blend it until smooth and transfer in the mixing bowl. Add minced garlic, Feta cheese, ground paprika, eggs, and diced onion. Mix up well. Place the spinach mixture in the casserole mold and flatten it well. Cover the spinach mixture with remaining Phyllo dough and pour remaining butter over it. Bake spanakopita for 1 hour at 350F. Cut it into the servings.

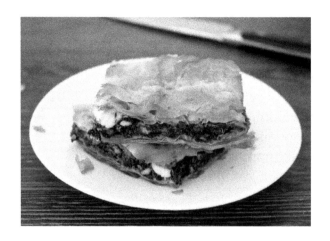

Notes:

18. Overnight Oats with Nuts

INGREDIENTS (4 Servings)

- ½ cup oats
- 2 teaspoons chia seeds, dried
- 1 tablespoon almond, chopped
- ½ teaspoon walnuts, chopped
- 1 cup skim milk 2 teaspoons honey
- ½ teaspoon vanilla extract

DIRECTIONS (8 hours 10 minutes)

In the big bowl mix up together chia seeds, oats, honey, and vanilla extract. Then add skim milk, walnuts, and almonds. Stir well. Transfer the prepared mixture into the mason jars and close with lids. Put the mason jars in the fridge and leave overnight. Store the meal in the fridge up to 2 days.

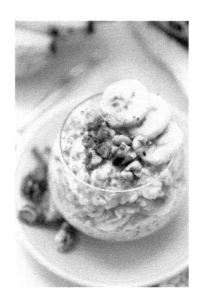

Notes:

19. Poblano Fritatta

- 5 eggs, beaten
- 1 poblano chile, chopped, raw
- 1 oz scallions, chopped
- 1/3 cup heavy cream
- ½ teaspoon butter
- ½ teaspoon salt
- ½ teaspoon chili flakes
- 1 tablespoon fresh cilantro, chopped

DIRECTIONS (25 minutes)

Mix up together eggs with heavy cream and whisk until homogenous. Add chopped poblano chile, scallions, salt, chili flakes, and fresh cilantro. Toss butter in the skillet and melt it. Add egg mixture and flatten it in the skillet if needed. Close the lid and cook the frittata for 15 minutes over the medium-low heat. When the frittata is cooked, it will be solid.

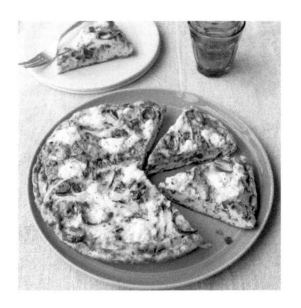

Notes:

20. Vegetable Breakfast Bowl

- 1 cup sweet potatoes, peeled, chopped
- 1 russet potato, chopped
- 1 red onion, sliced
- 2 bell pepper, trimmed
- ½ teaspoon garlic powder
- ¾ teaspoon onion powder
- 1 tablespoon olive oil
- 1 tablespoon Sriracha sauce
- 1 tablespoon coconut milk

DIRECTIONS (45 minutes)

Line the baking tray with baking paper. Place the chopped russet potato and sweet potato in the tray. Add onion, bell peppers, and sprinkle the vegetables with olive oil, onion powder, and garlic powder. Mix up the vegetables well with the help of the fingertips and transfer in the preheated to the 360F oven. Bake the vegetables for 45 minutes. Meanwhile, make the sauce: mix up together Sriracha sauce and coconut milk. Transfer the cooked vegetables in the serving plates and sprinkle with Sriracha sauce.

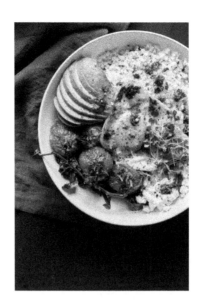

Notes:

21. Simple and Quick Steak

- ½ lb steak, quality
- cut Salt and freshly cracked black pepper

DIRECTIONS (25 minutes)

Switch on the air fryer, set frying basket in it, then set its temperature to 385°F and let preheat. Meanwhile, prepare the steaks, and for this, season steaks with salt and freshly cracked black pepper on both sides. When air fryer has preheated, add prepared steaks in the fryer basket, shut it with lid and cook for 15 minutes. When done, transfer steaks to a dish and then serve immediately. For meal prepping, evenly divide the steaks between two heatproof containers, close them with lid and refrigerate for up to 3 days until ready to serve. When ready to eat, reheat steaks into the microwave until hot and then serve.

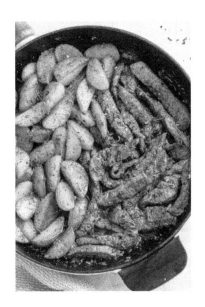

Notes:

22. Cheesy Eggs in Avocado

- 1 medium avocado
- 2 organic eggs
- ¼ cup shredded cheddar cheese
- Salt and freshly cracked black pepper
- 1 tbsp olive oil

DIRECTIONS (35 minutes)

Switch on the oven, then set its temperature to 425°F, and let preheat. Meanwhile, prepare the avocados and for this, cut the avocado in half and remove its pit. Take two muffin tins, grease them with oil, and then add an avocado half into each tin. Crack an egg into each avocado half, season well with salt and freshly cracked black pepper, and then sprinkle cheese on top. When the oven has preheated, place the muffin tins in the oven and bake for 15 minutes until cooked. When done, take out the muffin tins, transfer the avocados baked organic eggs to a dish, and then serve them.

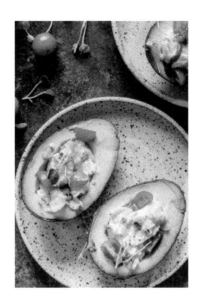

Notes:

23. Four-Cheese Zucchini Noodles with Basil Pesto

- 4 cups zucchini noodles
- 4 oz Mascarpone cheese
- 1/8 cup Romano cheese
- 2 tbsp grated parmesan cheese
- ¼ tsp salt
- ½ tsp cracked black pepper
- 2 1/8 tsp ground nutmeg
- 1/8 cup basil pesto
- ½ cup shredded mozzarella cheese
- 1 tbsp olive oil

DIRECTIONS (25 minutes)

Switch on the oven, then set its temperature to 400°F and let it preheat. Meanwhile, place zucchini noodles in a heatproof bowl and microwave at high heat setting for 3 minutes, set aside until required. Take another heatproof bowl, add all cheeses in it, except for mozzarella, season with salt, black pepper and nutmeg, and microwave at high heat setting for 1 minute until cheese has melted. Whisk the cheese mixture, add cooked zucchini noodles in it along with basil pesto and mozzarella cheese and fold until well mixed. Take a casserole dish, grease it with oil, add zucchini noodles mixture in it, and then bake for 10 minutes until done. Serve straight away.

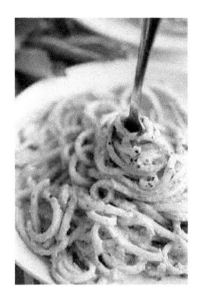

Notes:

24. Heavenly Egg Bake with Blackberry

- Chopped rosemary
- 1 tsp lime zest
- ½ tsp salt
- ¼ tsp vanilla extract, unsweetened
- 1 tsp grated ginger
- 3 tbsp coconut flour
- 1 tbsp unsalted butter
- 5 organic eggs
- 1 tbsp olive oil
- ½ cup fresh blackberries
- Black pepper to taste

DIRECTIONS (25 minutes)

Switch on the oven, then set its temperature to 350°F and let it preheat. Meanwhile, place all the ingredients in a blender, reserving the berries and pulse for 2 to 3 minutes until well blended and smooth. Take four silicon muffin cups, grease them with oil, evenly distribute the blended batter in the cups, top with black pepper and bake for 15 minutes until cooked through and the top has golden brown. When done, let blueberry egg bake cool in the muffin cups for 5 minutes, then take them out, cool them on a wire rack and then serve. For meal prepping, wrap each egg bake with aluminum foil and freeze for up to 3 days. When ready to eat, reheat blueberry egg bake in the microwave and then serve.

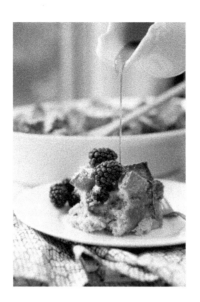

Notes:

25. Blueberry and Vanilla Scones

- 1½ cup almond flour
- 3 organic eggs, beaten
- 2 tsp baking powder
- ½ cup stevia
- 2 tsp vanilla extract, unsweetened
- ¾ cup fresh raspberries
- 1 tbsp olive oil

DIRECTIONS (20 minutes)

Switch on the oven, then set its temperature to 375 °F and let it preheat. Take a large bowl, add flour and eggs in it, stir in baking powder, stevia, and vanilla until combined and then fold in berries until mixed. Take a baking dish, grease it with oil, scoop the prepared batter on it with an ice cream scoop and bake for 10 minutes until done. When done, transfer scones on a wire rack, cool them completely, and then serve.

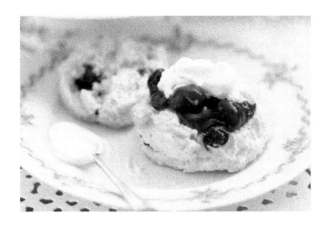

Notes:

26. Avocado and Eggs Breakfast Tacos

INGREDIENTS (2 Servings)

- 4 organic eggs
- 1 tbsp unsalted butter
- 2 low-carb tortillas
- 2 tbsp mayonnaise
- 4 sprigs of cilantro
- ½ of an avocado, sliced
- Salt and freshly cracked black pepper, to taste
- 1 tbsp Tabasco sauce

DIRECTIONS (23 minutes)

Take a bowl, crack eggs in it and whisk well until smooth. Take a skillet pan, place it over medium heat, add butter and when it melts, pour in eggs, spread them evenly in the pan and cook for 4 to 5 minutes until done. When done, transfer eggs to a plate and set aside until required. Add tortillas into the pan, cook for 2 to 3 minutes per side until warm through, and then transfer them onto a plate. Assemble tacos and for this, spread mayonnaise on the side of each tortilla, then distribute cooked eggs, and top with cilantro and sliced avocado. Season with salt and black pepper, drizzle with tabasco sauce, and roll up the tortillas. Serve straight away or store in the refrigerator for up to 2 days until ready to eat.

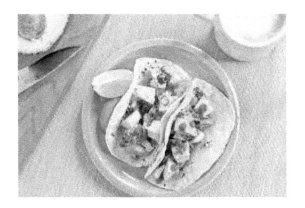

Notes:

27. Awesome Coffee with Butter

- 1 cup of water
- 1 tbsp coconut oil
- 1 tbsp unsalted butter
- 2 tbsp coffee

DIRECTIONS (10 minutes)

Take a small pan, place it over medium heat, pour in water, and bring to boil. Then add remaining ingredients, stir well, and cook until butter and oil have melted. Remove pan from heat, pass the coffee through a strainer, and serve immediately.

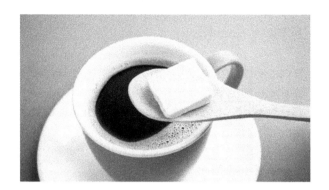

Notes:

28. Cheesy Caprese Style Portobellos Mushrooms

INGREDIENTS (4 Servings)

- 2 large caps of Portobello mushroom, gills removed
- 4 tomatoes, halved
- Salt and freshly cracked black pepper, to taste
- ¼ cup fresh basil
- 4 tbsp olive oil
- ¼ cup shredded Mozzarella cheese

DIRECTIONS (20 minutes)

Switch on the oven, then set its temperature to 400°F and let it preheat. Meanwhile, prepare mushrooms, and for this, brush them with olive oil and set aside until required. Place tomatoes in a bowl, season with salt and black pepper, add basil, drizzle with oil and toss until mixed. Distribute cheese evenly in the bottom of each mushroom cap and then top with prepared tomato mixture. Take a baking sheet, line it with aluminum foil, place prepared mushrooms on it and bake for 15 minutes until thoroughly cooked. Serve straight away.

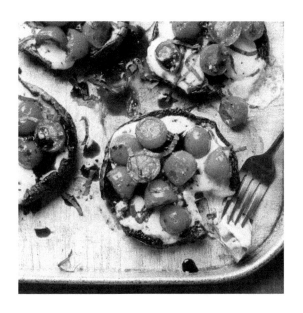

Notes:

29. Scrambled Eggs

- 1 tablespoon butter
- 4 eggs
- Salt and black pepper, to taste

DIRECTIONS (25 minutes)

Combine together eggs, salt and black pepper in a bowl and keep aside. Heat butter in a pan over medium-low heat and slowly add the whisked eggs. Stir the eggs continuously in the pan with the help of a fork for about 4 minutes. Dish out in a plate and serve immediately. You can refrigerate this scramble for about 2 days for meal prepping and reuse by heating it in microwave oven.

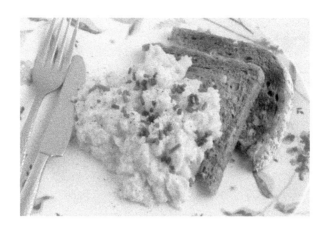

Notes:

30. Creamy Parsley Soufflé

INGREDIENTS (2 Servings)

- 2 fresh red chili peppers, chopped
- Salt, to taste
- 4 eggs
- 4 tablespoons light cream
- 2 tablespoons fresh parsley, chopped

DIRECTIONS (25 minutes)

Preheat the oven to 375 degrees F and grease 2 soufflé dishes. Combine all the ingredients in a bowl and mix well. Put the mixture into prepared soufflé dishes and transfer in the oven. Cook for about 6 minutes and dish out to serve immediately. For meal prepping, you can refrigerate this creamy parsley soufflé in the ramekins covered in a foil for about 2-3 days.

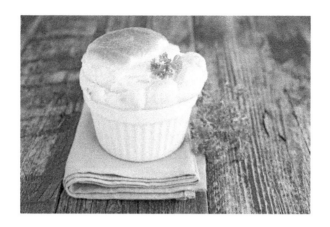

Notes:

31. Spinach Artichoke Egg Casserole

- 1/8 cup milk
- 2.5-ounce frozen chopped spinach, thawed and drained well
- 1/8 cup parmesan cheese
- 1/8 cup onions, shaved
- ¼ teaspoon salt
- ¼ teaspoon crushed red pepper
- 4 large eggs
- 3.5-ounce artichoke hearts, drained
- ¼ cup white cheddar, shredded
- 1/8 cup ricotta cheese
- ½ garlic clove, minced
- ¼ teaspoon dried thyme

DIRECTIONS (45 minutes)

Preheat the oven to 350 degrees F and grease a baking dish with non-stick cooking spray. Whisk eggs and milk together and add artichoke hearts and spinach. Mix well and stir in rest of the ingredients, withholding the ricotta cheese. Pour the mixture into the baking dish and top evenly with ricotta cheese. Transfer in the oven and bake for about 30 minutes. Dish out and serve warm.

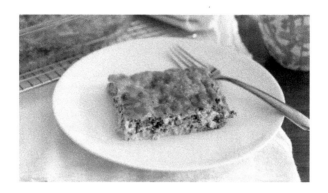

Notes:

32. Cinnamon Faux-St Crunch Cereal

INGREDIENTS (2 Servings)

- ¼ cup hulled hemp seeds
- ½ tablespoon coconut oil
- ¼ cup milled flax seed
- 1 tablespoon ground cinnamon
- ¼ cup apple juice

DIRECTIONS (35 minutes)

Preheat the oven to 300 degrees F and line a cookie sheet with parchment paper. Put hemp seeds, flax seed and ground cinnamon in a food processor. Add coconut oil and apple juice and blend until smooth. Pour the mixture on the cookie sheet and transfer in the oven. Bake for about 15 minutes and lower the temperature of the oven to 250 degrees F. Bake for another 10 minutes and dish out from the oven, turning it off. Cut into small squares and place in the turned off oven. Place the cereal in the oven for 1 hour until it is crisp. Dish out and serve with unsweetened almond milk.

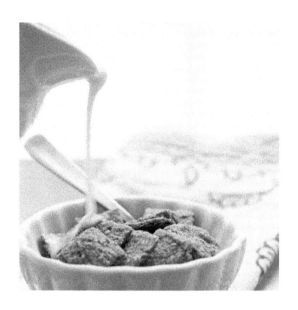

Notes:

33. Keto Egg Fast Snickerdoodle Crepes

- 5 oz cream cheese, softened
- 6 eggs
- 1 teaspoon cinnamon
- Butter, for frying
- 1 tablespoon Swerve
- 2 tablespoons granulated Swerve
- 8 tablespoons butter, softened
- 1 tablespoon cinnamon

DIRECTIONS (15 minutes)

For the crepes: Put all the ingredients together in a blender except the butter and process until smooth. Heat butter on medium heat in a non-stick pan and pour some batter in the pan. Cook for about 2 minutes, then flip and cook for 2 more minutes. Repeat with the remaining mixture. Mix Swerve, butter and cinnamon in a small bowl until combined. Spread this mixture onto the centre of the crepe and serve rolled up.

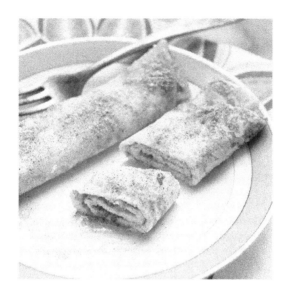

Notes:

34. Oat & Carrot Cupcakes

- 1 ½ cups grated carrots
- ¼ cup pecans, chopped
- 1 cup oat bran
- 1 cup wholewheat flour
- ½ cup all-purpose flour
- ½ cup old-fashioned oats
- 3 tbsp light brown sugar
- 1 tsp vanilla extract
- ½ lemon, zested
- 1 tsp baking powder
- 2 tsp ground cinnamon
- 2 tsp ground ginger
- ½ tsp ground nutmeg
- ¼ tsp salt
- 1¼ cups soy milk
- 2 tbsp honey
- 1 egg
- 2 tbsp olive oil

DIRECTIONS (30 minutes)

Preheat oven to 350 F and grease two lined with paper muffin tins with cooking spray. Mix whole-wheat flour, all-purpose flour, oat bran, oats, sugar, baking powder, cinnamon, nutmeg, ginger, and salt in a bowl; set aside. Beat egg with soy milk, honey, vanilla, lemon zest, and olive oil in another bowl. Pour this mixture into the flour mixture and combine to blend, leaving some lumps. Stir in carrots and pecans. Spoon batter into each coated muffin cup 3/4 way up. Bake for about 20 minutes. Prick with a toothpick and if it comes out easily, the cakes are cooked done. Let cool and serve.

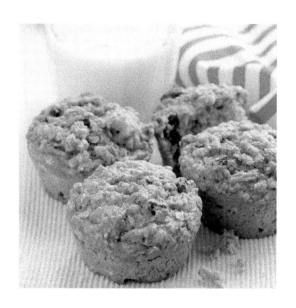

Notes:

35. Mushroom & Cherry Tomato Frittata

- 1 cup Italian brown mushrooms, sliced
- 2 spring onions, chopped
- 8 cherry tomatoes, halved
- 6 eggs
- ½ cup milk Salt and black pepper to taste
- 2 tbsp olive oil
- ¼ cup grated Parmesan cheese
- ½ tbsp Italian seasoning mix

DIRECTIONS (28 minutes)

Preheat oven to 370 F. Mix eggs, milk, Italian seasoning, salt, and pepper in a bowl. Warm olive oil in a skillet over medium heat until sizzling. Add in mushrooms, spring onions, and tomatoes and sauté for 5 minutes. Pour in the egg mixture and cook for 5 minutes until the eggs are set. Scatter Parmesan cheese and bake in the oven for 6-7 minutes until the cheese melts. Slice before serving.

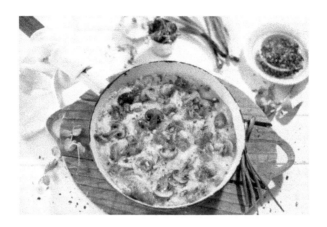

Notes:

36. Strawberry-Chocolate Smoothie

- 1 cup buttermilk
- 2 cups strawberries, hulled
- 1 cup crushed ice
- 3 tbsp cocoa powder
- 3 tbsp honey
- 2 mint leaves

DIRECTIONS (5 minutes)

In a food processor, pulse buttermilk, strawberries, ice, cocoa powder, mint, and honey until smooth. Serve.

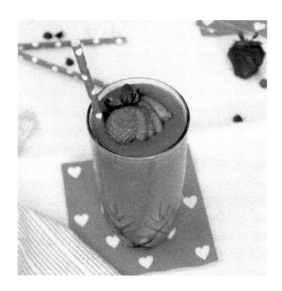

Notes:

37. Yogurt Parfait with Berries & Granola

- 2 cups berries
- 1 ½ cups Greek yogurt
- 1 tbsp powdered sugar
- ¼ cup granola

DIRECTIONS (5 minutes)

Divide between two bowls a layer of berries, yogurt, and powdered sugar. Scatter with granola and serve.

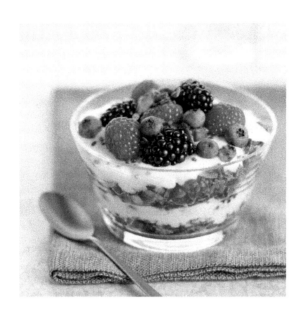

Notes:

38. Cheesy Cauliflower Frittata

INGREDIENTS (4 Servings)

- 2 tbsp olive oil
- ½ lb cauliflower florets
- ½ cup skimmed milk
- 6 eggs
- 1 red bell pepper, seeded and chopped
- ½ cup fontina cheese, grated
- ½ tsp red pepper
- ½ tsp turmeric Salt and black pepper to taste

DIRECTIONS (30 minutes)

Preheat oven to 360 F. In a bowl, beat the eggs with milk. Add in fontina cheese, red pepper, turmeric, salt, and pepper. Mix in red bell pepper. Warm olive oil in a skillet over medium heat and pour in the egg mixture; cook for 4-5 minutes. Set aside. Blanch the cauliflower florets in a pot for 5 minutes until tender. Spread over the egg mixture. Place the skillet in the oven and bake for 15 minutes or until it is set and golden brown. Allow cooling for a few minutes before slicing. Serve sliced.

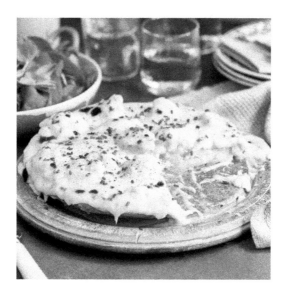

Notes:

39. Coconut & Chocolate Porridge with Bananas

INGREDIENTS (4 Servings)

- 2 bananas
- 4 dried apricots, chopped
- 1 cup barley, soaked overnight
- 2 tbsp flax seeds
- 1 tbsp cocoa powder
- 1 cup coconut milk
- ¼ tsp mint leaves
- 2 oz dark chocolate bars, grated
- 2 tbsp coconut flakes

DIRECTIONS (20 minutes)

Place the barley in a saucepan along with the flaxseeds and two cups of water. Bring to a boil, then lower the heat and simmer for 12 minutes, stirring often. Meanwhile, in a food processor, blend bananas, cocoa powder, coconut milk, apricots, and mint leaves until smooth. Once the barley is ready, stir in chocolate. Add in banana mixture. Spoon into bowls and garnish with coconut flakes. Serve.

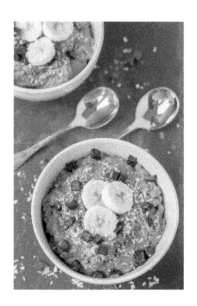

Notes:

40. Cilantro Mozzarella & Olive Cakes

INGREDIENTS (6 Servings)

- ¼ cup mozzarella cheese, shredded
- ¼ cup black olives, pitted and chopped
- ½ cup low-fat milk
- 4 tbsp coconut oil, softened
- 1 egg, beaten
- 1 cup cornflour
- 1 tsp baking powder
- 3 sun-dried tomatoes, finely chopped
- 2 tbsp fresh parsley, chopped
- 2 tbsp fresh cilantro, chopped
- ¼ tsp kosher salt

DIRECTIONS (25 minutes)

Preheat oven to 360 F. In a bowl, whisk the egg with milk and coconut oil. In a separate bowl, mix the salt, cornflour, cilantro, and baking powder. Combine the wet ingredients with the dry mixture. Stir in black olives, tomatoes, herbs, and mozzarella cheese. Pour the mixture into greased ramekins and bake for around 18-20 minutes or until cooked and golden.

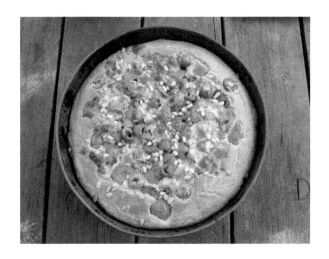

Notes:

41. Cheddar Egg Sandwich with Veggies

INGREDIENTS (2 Servings)

- 2 slices fontina cheese, crumbled
- 1 tbsp olive oil
- 3 eggs
- 1 tbsp butter
- 4 slices multigrain bread
- 1 Iceberg lettuce, separated into leaves
- 3 radishes, sliced
- ½ cucumber, sliced
- 2 pimiento peppers, seeded and chopped
- Salt and red pepper to taste

DIRECTIONS (15 minutes)

Warm the oil in a skillet over medium heat. Crack in the eggs and cook until the whites are set. Season with salt and red pepper; remove to a plate. Brush the bread slices with the butter and toast them in the same skillet for 2 minutes per side. Arrange 3 bread slices on a flat surface and put over the eggs. Add in the remaining ingredients and top with the remaining slices. Serve immediately.

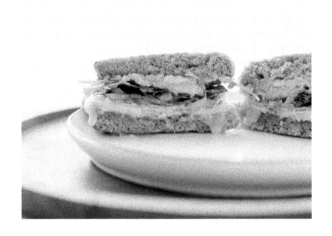

Notes:

42. Mushroom & Quinoa Cups

- 6 eggs
- 1 cup quinoa, cooked
- Salt and black pepper to taste
- 1 cup Gruyere cheese, grated
- 1 small yellow onion, chopped
- 1 cup mushrooms, sliced
- ½ cup green olives, chopped

DIRECTIONS (40 minutes)

Beat the eggs, salt, pepper, Gruyere cheese, onion, mushrooms, and green olives in a bowl. Pour into a silicone muffin tray and bake for 30 minutes at 360 F. Serve warm.

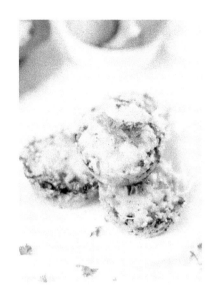

Notes:

43. Raspberry Oat Pudding

- 1 cup almond milk
- ½ cup rolled oats
- 1 tbsp flax seeds
- 2 tsp honey
- 1 cup raspberries, pureed
- 1 tbsp yogurt

DIRECTIONS (5 minutes)

Toss the oats, almond milk, chia seeds, honey, and raspberries in a bowl. Serve in bowls topped with yogurt.

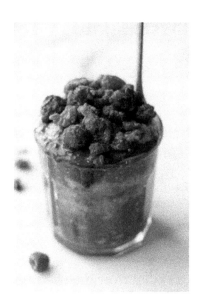

Notes:

44. Classic Spanish Tortilla

INGREDIENTS (4 Servings)

- 1 ½ lb gold potatoes, peeled and sliced
- 1 sweet onion, thinly sliced
- 8 eggs
- ½ dried oregano
- ½ cup olive oil
- Salt to taste

DIRECTIONS (35 minutes)

Heat the olive oil in a skillet over medium heat. Fry the potatoes for 8-10 minutes, stirring often. Add in onion and salt and cook for 5-6 minutes until the potatoes are tender and slightly golden; set aside. In a bowl, beat the eggs with a pinch of salt. Add in the potato mixture and mix well. Pour into the skillet and cook for about 10-12 minutes. Flip the tortilla using a plate, and cook for 2 more minutes until nice and crispy. Slice and serve warm.

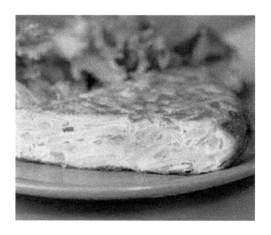

Notes:

45. Easy Onion-Mushroom Omelet

- 1 Granny Smith apple, chopped
- 2 cups spinach
- 1 avocado, peeled, pitted and chopped
- 1 tsp honey
- 2 cups almond milk

DIRECTIONS (5 minutes)

Place spinach, apple, avocado, honey, and almond milk in a food processor and blend until smooth. Serve chilled.

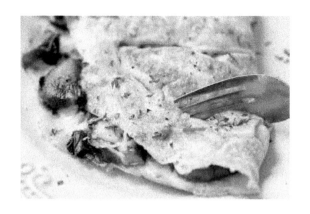

Notes:

46. Zucchini & Mushroom Egg Cakes

- 1 cup Parmesan cheese, grated
- 1 onion, chopped
- 1 cup mushrooms, sliced
- 1 red bell pepper, chopped
- 1 zucchini, chopped
- Salt and black pepper to taste
- 8 eggs, whisked
- 1 tbsp olive oil
- 2 tbsp chives, chopped

DIRECTIONS (20 minutes)

Preheat the oven to 360 F. Warm the olive oil in a skillet over medium heat and sauté onion, zucchini, mushrooms, salt, and pepper for 5 minutes until tender. Distribute the mixture across muffin cups and top with the eggs. Sprinkle with salt, pepper, and chives and bake for 10 minutes. Serve immediately.

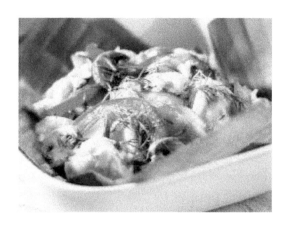

Notes:

47. Egg & Zucchini Stuffed Tomatoes

INGREDIENTS (4 Servings)

- 2 tbsp olive oil
- ¼ cup milk
- 1 small zucchini, chopped
- 8 tomatoes, insides scooped
- 8 eggs
- ¼ cup Parmesan cheese, grated
- Salt and black pepper to taste
- 2 tbsp rosemary, chopped

DIRECTIONS (25 minutes)

Preheat the oven to 360 F. Place tomatoes on a greased baking dish. Mix the zucchini with milk, salt, and pepper. Divide the mixture between the tomatoes and crack an egg on each one. Top with Parmesan cheese and rosemary and bake in the oven for 15 minutes. Serve hot.

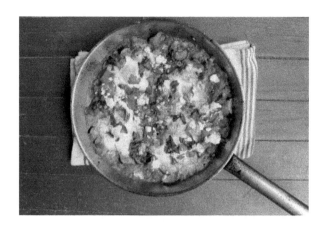

Notes:

48. Anchovy Egg Scramble

INGREDIENTS (4 Servings)

- 2 tbsp olive oil
- 1 green bell pepper, chopped
- 2 anchovy fillets, chopped
- 8 cherry tomatoes, cubed
- 2 spring onions, chopped
- 1 tbsp capers, drained
- 5 black olives, pitted and sliced
- 6 eggs, beaten
- Salt and black pepper to taste
- ¼ tsp dried oregano
- 1 tbsp parsley, chopped

DIRECTIONS (20 minutes)

Warm the olive oil in a skillet over medium heat and cook the bell pepper and spring onions for 3 minutes. Add in anchovies, cherry tomatoes, capers, and black olives and cook for another 2 minutes. Stir in eggs and sprinkle with salt, pepper, and oregano and scramble for 5 minutes. Serve sprinkled with parsley.

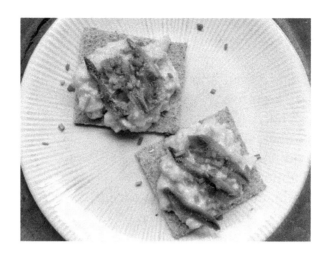

Notes:

49. Watercress & Egg Salad with Quinoa

- 2 boiled eggs, cut into wedges
- 2 cups watercress
- 2 cups cherry tomatoes, halved
- 1 cucumber, sliced
- 1 cup quinoa, cooked
- 1 cup almonds, chopped
- 1 avocado, peeled, pitted and sliced
- 2 tbsp fresh cilantro, chopped
- Salt to taste
- 1 lemon, juiced

DIRECTIONS (5 minutes)

Place watercress, cherry tomatoes, cucumber, quinoa, almonds, olive oil, cilantro, salt, and lemon juice in a bowl and toss to combine. Top with egg wedges and avocado slices and serve immediately.

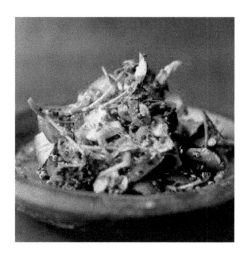

Notes:

50. Vegetable Egg Bake

- ½ cup whole milk
- 8 eggs
- 1 cup spinach, chopped
- 4 oz canned artichokes, chopped
- 1 garlic clove, minced
- ½ cup Parmesan cheese, crumbled
- 1 tsp oregano, dried
- 1 tsp Jalapeño pepper, minced
- Salt to taste
- 2 tsp olive oil

DIRECTIONS (55 minutes)

Preheat oven to 360 F. Warm the olive oil in a skillet over medium heat and sauté garlic and spinach for 3 minutes. Beat the eggs in a bowl. Stir in artichokes, milk, Parmesan cheese, oregano, jalapeño pepper, and salt. Add in spinach mixture and toss to combine. Transfer to a greased baking dish and bake for 20 minutes until golden and bubbling. Slice into wedges and serve.

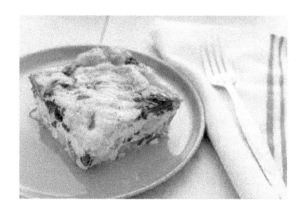

Notes:

51. Awesome Tuna Salad

INGREDIENTS (2 Servings)

- ½ iceberg lettuce, torn
- ¼ endive, chopped
- 1 tomato, cut into wedges
- 2 tbsp olive oil
- 5 oz canned tuna in water, flaked
- 4 black olives, pitted and sliced
- 1 tbsp lemon juice
- Salt and black pepper to taste

DIRECTIONS (10 minutes)

In a salad bowl, mix olive oil, lemon juice, salt, and pepper. Add in lettuce, endive, and tuna and toss to coat. Top with black olives and tomato wedges and serve.

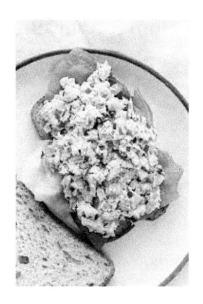

Notes:

52. Shrimp & Avocado Salad

INGREDIENTS (4 Servings)

- 2 tbsp olive oil
- 1 tbsp lemon juice
- 1 yellow bell pepper, sliced
- 1 Romano lettuce, torn
- 1 avocado, chopped Salt to taste
- 1 lb shrimp, peeled and deveined
- 1 cups cherry tomatoes, halved

DIRECTIONS (10 minutes)

Preheat grill pan over high heat. Drizzle the shrimp with some olive oil and arrange them on the preheated grill pan. Sear for 5 minutes on both sides until pink and cooked through. Let cool completely. In a serving plate, arrange the lettuce, and top with bell pepper, shrimp, avocado, and cherry tomatoes. In a bowl, add the lemon juice, salt, and olive oil and whisk to combine. Drizzle the dressing over the salad and serve immediately.

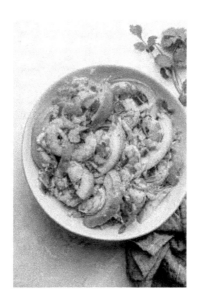

Notes:

53. One-Pan Eggplant Quinoa

- 2 tbsp olive oil
- 1 shallot, chopped
- 2 garlic cloves, minced
- 1 tomato, chopped
- 1 cup quinoa
- 1 eggplant, cubed
- 2 tbsp basil, chopped
- ¼ cup green olives, pitted and chopped
- ½ cup feta cheese, crumbled
- 1 cup canned garbanzo beans, drained and rinsed
- Salt and black pepper to taste

DIRECTIONS (30 minutes)

Warm the olive oil in a skillet over medium heat and sauté garlic, shallot, and eggplant for 4-5 minutes until tender. Pour in quinoa and 2 cups of water. Season with salt and pepper and bring to a boil. Reduce the heat to low and cook for 15 minutes.Stir in olives, feta cheese, and garbanzo beans. Serve topped with basil.

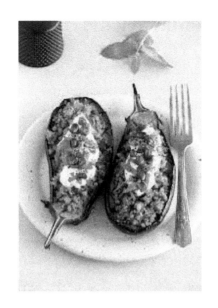

Notes:

54. Arugula & Gorgonzola Salad

- 3 tbsp olive oil
- 1 cucumber, cubed
- 15 oz canned garbanzo beans, drained
- 3 oz black olives, pitted and sliced
- 1 Roma tomato, slivered
- ¼ cup red onion, chopped
- 5 cups arugula Salt to taste
- ½ cup Gorgonzola cheese, crumbled
- 1 tbsp lemon juice
- 2 tbsp parsley, chopped

DIRECTIONS (10 minutes)

Place the arugula in a salad bowl. Add in garbanzo beans, cucumber, olives, tomato, and onion and mix to combine. In another small bowl, whisk the lemon juice, olive oil, and salt. Drizzle the dressing over the salad and sprinkle with gorgonzola cheese to serve.

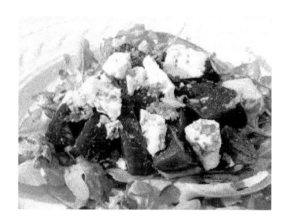

Notes:

55. Greek-Style Pasta Salad

- 2 tbsp olive oil
- 16 oz fusilli pasta
- 1 yellow bell pepper, cubed
- 1 green bell pepper, cubed
- Salt and black pepper to taste
- 3 tomatoes, cubed
- 1 red onion, sliced
- 2 cups feta cheese, crumbled
- ¼ cup lemon juice
- 1 tbsp lemon zest, grated
- 1 cucumber, cubed
- 1 cup Kalamata olives, pitted and sliced

DIRECTIONS (10 minutes)

Cook the fusilli pasta in boiling salted water until "al dente", 8-10 minutes. Drain and set asite to cool. In a bowl, whisk together olive oil, lemon zst, lemon juice, and salt. Add in bell peppers, tomatoes, onion, feta cheese, cucumber, olives, and pasta and toss to combine. Serve immediately.

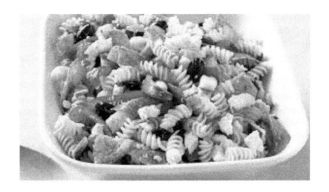

Notes:

56. Cheesy Thyme Waffles

- ½ cup mozzarella cheese, finely shredded
- ¼ cup Parmesan cheese
- ¼ large head cauliflower
- ½ cup collard greens
- 1 large egg
- 1 stalk green onion
- ½ tablespoon olive oil
- ½ teaspoon garlic powder
- ¼ teaspoon salt
- ½ tablespoon sesame seed
- 1 teaspoon fresh thyme, chopped
- ¼ teaspoon ground black pepper

DIRECTIONS (15 minutes)

Put cauliflower, collard greens, spring onion and thyme in a food processor and pulse until smooth. Dish out the mixture in a bowl and stir in rest of the ingredients. Heat a waffle iron and transfer the mixture evenly over the griddle. Cook until a waffle is formed and dish out in a serving platter.

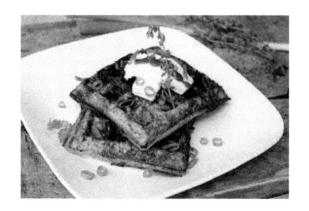

Notes:

57. Low Carb Green Smoothie

- 1/3 cup romaine lettuce
- 1/3 tablespoon fresh ginger, peeled and chopped
- 1½ cups filtered water
- 1/8 cup fresh pineapple, chopped
- ¾ tablespoon fresh parsley
- 1/3 cup raw cucumber, peeled and sliced
- ¼ Hass avocado
- ¼ cup kiwi fruit, peeled and chopped
- 1/3 tablespoon Swerve

DIRECTIONS (15 minutes)

Put all the ingredients in a blender and blend until smooth. Pour into 2 serving glasses and serve chilled.

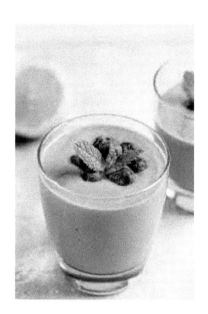

Notes:

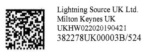

Lightning Source UK Ltd.
Milton Keynes UK
UKHW022020190421
382278UK00003B/524

9 781914 438899